YOUR KNOWLEDGE HAS VALUE

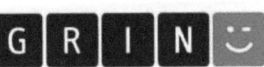

Fungal infestation of onion bulbs during storage in sack and on its antioxidant properties

Bamidele Ijigbade

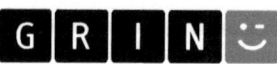

Bibliographic information published by the German National Library:

The German National Library lists this publication in the National Bibliography; detailed bibliographic data are available on the Internet at http://dnb.dnb.de.

ISBN: 9783346793393
This book is also available as an ebook.

© GRIN Publishing GmbH
Nymphenburger Straße 86
80636 München

Print and binding: Books on Demand GmbH, Norderstedt, Germany
Printed on acid-free paper from responsible sources.

The present work has been carefully prepared. Nevertheless, authors and publishers do not incur liability for the correctness of information, notes, links and advice as well as any printing errors.

GRIN web shop: https://www.grin.com/document/1312514

FUNGAL INFESTATION OF ONION BULBS DURING STORAGE IN SACK AND ON ITS ANTIOXIDANT PROPERTIES

ABSTRACT

The aim of this study is to determine fungal infestation of onion bulbs during storage in sack and on its antioxidant properties. The fungal infestation of onion bulbs during storage in sack shows that five (5) fungi each were isolated from the onion bulbs during storage in sack at day zero (0) and day seven (7) respectively while at day fourteen (14), six fungal infestation was isolated from the onion bulbs during storage in sack. A total of sixteen (16) fungi infested the onion bulbs during storage in sack. The fungi belong to four (5) genera and six (6) species of fungi infested the onion bulbs during storage in sack. *Aspersillus niger* and *Aspersillus flavus* were the most frequently isolated fungi with 31.25% each followed by *Fusarium oxysporum* and *Aspergillus fumigatus* with 12.50% each while *Penicillium chrysogenum* and *Rhizopus stolonifer* recorded 6.25% each. The antioxidant analysis of onion extract after storage in sack for 14 days recorded at all concentrations (0.5, 0.25, 0.125, 0.0625 and 0.03125 mg/ml), show that the antioxidant property of the onion extract at day zero (0) and day 7 was higher than that 14. The inhibition of free radical DPPH at day zero (0) and 7 were 29.92 %, 49.21%, 69.29%, 70.07% and 47.63% while at day 14, the percentage (%) of inhibition of free radical DPPH were 29.33 %, 49.02%, 69.01%, 69.77% and 47.21% .

Contents

1.0 INTRODUCTION

1.1 Background of the Study

The onion (*Allium cepa* L.) is an important vegetable crop in Nigeria based on consumption and economic value to farmers. The crop is grown for its bulbs which are used daily in every home for seasoning and flavouring of foods. Onion is a valuable ingredient in the diet due to its content of sugars, vitamins and minerals (Ole *et al.*, 2014). The crop is grown mainly in the north, during the dry season (October to April). The onion farmers in Nigeria almost always store, their onions after harvest for one to five months to ensure a continual supply through seasons when fresh produce is unavailable. Bulb rots are a common cause of onion loss during storage.

Fungi, especially moulds are important pathogens of fruits and a vegetables particularly under tropical and sub-tropical conditions (Adebayo and Diyaolu, 2013). The importance of storage rots includes reduction in the quantity and quality of onion which affects the market value (Dogondaji *et al.*, 2015). Other important consequence often overlooked, is mycotoxin contamination of the affected material (Muhammad *et al.*, 2014).

Biological effects attributed to onions have been commonly ascribed to the volatile sulfur-containing compounds, such as thiosulfinates, mainly responsible for the characteristic taste, aroma and lachrymatory effects (Krest *et al.*, 2012). These compounds are formed from cysteine sulfoxide precursors and the effect of the enzyme alliinase which is released from cell vacuoles when tissues are damaged (Ioku *et al.*, 2011). However, these volatile products are highly unstable and recently, attention has been focused on the effects of phenolic compounds, such as flavonoids, which are more stable (Fossen *et al.*, 2011). Onion is known for being a good natural source of

4

flavonoids mainly represented by the flavonols - quercetin and kaempferol, which are present as their glycosides.

About 15 different fungal species and 5 bacterial species are found responsible for the onion diseases in the storage and transit all over the world. The loss due to these diseases is considerable and may go up to 40% (Dimka and Onuegbu, 2010). In storage various diseases destroy the onions such as Black mould rot (*Aspergillus niger*), Blue mould rot (*Penicillium* spp.), *Fusarium* bulb rot (*Fusarium* spp.), Basal rot (*Fusarium moniliforme*), *Aspergillus* rot (*Aspergillus* spp.), Dry rot (*Macrophomina phasiolina*), Soft rot (*Erwinia* spp.), Smudge (*Colletotrichum circinans*), Grey neck rot (*Botrytis allii*), Green mold rot (*Penicillium* spp.),White rot (*Sclerotium cepivorum*) and Anthracnose (*Colletotrichum chardonianum*) (Dimka and Onuegbu, 2010). Among these, black mould rot (*A. niger*) is more severe in storage. *A. niger* and *A. flavus* infect onion at high temperature and high relative humidity. Whereas *Penicillium* spp. destroys onion at low temperature. Sometimes *Penicillium* spp. produces mycotoxin, Penitrem A, which has been previously implicated in tremorgenictoxicosis (Adebayo and Diyaolu, 2013). It is reported that the predominant fungal pathogens associated with the storage diseases of onions were *Aspergillus* sp., *Penicillium* sp. and *Fusarium* sp. (Adebayo and Diyaolu, 2013).

1.2 Aim of the Study
The aim of this study is to determine fungal infestation of onion bulbs during storage in sack and on its antioxidant properties.

1.3   Objectives of the Study

The specific objectives of the study are to:

i.   Assess fungal infestation of onion bulb during storage in sack

ii.   Identify the isolated fungi from onion bulbs stored in sack

iii.   Determine the antioxidant properties of the onion bulbs stored in sack

2.0   LITERATURE REVIEW

2.1   Uses of *Allium cepa*

Allium cepa has been traditionally used for its remedial characteristics in the management of

various ailments. The essence of *A. cepa* proliferated into ancient Greece where it was used as a

blood purifier for athletes. During the invasion of Rome, gladiators used to rub down onion juice

to firm up the muscles. The Greek and Phoenicians sailors consumed it to prevent scurvy.

Moreover, the Greek physician Hippocrates, used to prescribe onion as a wound healer, diuretic

and pneumonia fighters. In the 6th century, onion was described as one of the indispensable

vegetable or spice and medicine (Kabrah 2010). *A. cepa* was most regularly used in low developed

countries. This could be probably due to the lack of medical facilities and the easy availability of

traditional remedies including onion. *A. cepa* is commonly taken raw or as a decoction for treating

infectious diseases. It is also used in a wide variety of preparations for internal and external use to

relieve several ailments including digestive problems, skin diseases, metabolic disease, insect bites

and others (Silambarasan and Ayyanar 2015).

2.2   Post-harvest losses in onion

Storage is one of the important aspects for post-harvest handling of onion. The storage condition

extends the period of availability of fresh onion by arresting the metabolic breakdown and decay.

It is achieved by controlling the Relative humidity and Temperature. The storage life of onion is depending on different parameter such as Physiological activity, Biochemical activity and Microbial invasion. Inadequate and improper field curing after harvest, infection by different pathogen, sprouting and also poor storage methods being practiced by the farmers are the main reasons of prevailing losses. In general, the losses due to reduction in weight, sprouting and rotting (decay) were found to be 20-25, 4-5, and 10-12 % respectively (Jaradat et al. 2016). Currently about 35- 40 %of the onion is estimated to be lost as postharvest losses during various post- harvest operations including handling and storage (Akash et al., 2014). Onion suffers from many diseases from pre harvest to post harvest period. The survey conducted at the international level revealed that about 35-40% onion is lost due to damage caused by different diseases (Gupta et al., 2010). A number of microorganisms are responsible for bulb rotting of onion, but among them, fungi are the main causal agent responsible for pre and post-harvest period losses in the onion (Hayta et al. 2014). It makes it prone to the development of various fungal pathogens of different genera and species and in turn leading to the damage by causing rot during the storage. Identification of pathogens which causes diseases in onion is essential for effective inhibition of target pathogens. Various species of *Aspergillus* pathogens are reported to cause blue mould on onion bulb during storage. The blue moulds are frequently isolated from stored diseased bulbs of local cultivars of onion (Sharma et al. 2014). *Aspergillus niger* is able to produce mycotoxin which reduces the quality and quantity of food products and feed-stuff which is a potent hepatic- carcinogen in humans and animals (Irkin and Korukluoglu, 2017). The fungus causing black mold is the main member of *Aspergillus* and is predominantly a plant pathogen responsible for post-harvest deterioration of stored food materials (Kocic-Tanackov et al., 2019).It is responsible for the deterioration of agricultural product during pre and post-harvest stages. It affects the availability

7

of onion to domestic and international trade. The infestation of fungi causes spoilage and ultimately decreases the qualitative attributes and quantity of food (Liguori *et al.*, 2017).Being saprophytic and filamentous in morphology *Aspergillus niger* resides and perpetuates in soil, forage, organic debris and food products causing black mold disease during post-harvest stage of onion bulbs (Kocic-Tanackov *et al.*, 2019). The most favourable temperature conditions for the growth of the fungus is 28°C-34°C followed by the warm and moist conditions eliciting infection (Liguori *et al.*, 2017). The contamination of pathogens begins at germination stage and remains up till storage period (Ferreres *et al.*, 2010). The pathogen transmission is by infected soil or seed and the infected bulbs shows neck discoloration along with black coloured mycelia and the hiding spores in the outer dry scales (Corzo-Mart *et al.*, 2017).Chemical treatment is found best to inhibit Black mold and other fungal pathogens disease in the onion bulbs (Begum and Yassen, 2015).

2.3   Microorganisms Associated with Onion Spoilage in Nigeria

Onions are associated with micro-organisms which are capable of causing spoilage. This spoilage usually occurs during harvesting, post-harvesting, transportation, marketing and storage. In tropical countries the storage is in ambient temperature (24-32°c) and at a variable relative humidity depending on location and season.

Bulb-rot is a common cause of onion loss or spoilage during storage. They are caused by microorganisms particularly fungi the black mould disease caused by *Aspergillus niger* is a limiting factor in onion production worldwide. *Aspergillus niger* has been reported to survive between onion crops as a soil saprophyte in or on bulbs in field or storage and is ubiquitous in nature. Onions are prone to spoilage by fungi during harvesting, handing storing and marketing processes.

Adebayo and Diyaolu (2013) and Gashua *et al.* (2014) opined that fungi, especially moulds are important pathogens of fruits and vegetables particularly under tropical and sub-tropical condition. Gent and Mohan (2016) estimated that bulb rot account for 10%-15% of storage losses of different varieties during three-month storage period under local condition. Five fungal belonging to different genera are found to be responsible for the spoilage of onion bulbs. These genera include *Penicilum* spp., *Aspergillus flavus*, *Fusarium* spp, *Aspergillus niger* and *Mucor* spp. Among the fungi isolated from rotten bulbs, *Fusarium* species are responsible. *Aspergillus* spp grow on the surface of onion bulbs but did not cause rotting when inoculated artificially. Generally, spoilage fungi are known to toxigenic or pathogenic under favorable conditions (Adebayo *et al.*, 2012). Al-Hindi *et al.* (2011) isolated toxigenic fungi from spoiling fruit, pathogenic fungi are cable of causing infections. *Aspergillus* spp are known to produce several toxic metabolites.

During refrigeration some moulds may also produce mycotoxins. Bulb rottening by storage losses of onions in Nigeria as well as other countries in the world are well documented by Adamick (2014).

Botrytis Neck rot is also a microorganisms capable of causing spoilage in onion his is cause by *botrytis alli*, a fungus that over winter on plant debris in soil, on infected bulbs, and as sclerotia in soil. Economic effect on the economy of the onion bulbs farmers in the particular and the economy of the country in general. The control of the fungal spoilage of onion bulbs is therefore inevitable. Proper storage conditions, careful harvesting, protection of the bulbs from sunburn, provision of adequate ventilation and regular examination during storage will minimize the entry and proliferation of these organisms in the onion bulbs, thereby reducing the incidence of diseases cause by fungi and also improve the economy by reducing waste resulting from spoilage. Bacteria are of only minor important in the market spoilage of most vegetables e.g onions because of the acid PH value. The soft rot coliform bacteria, *Erwinia carotovara* and *Pseudomonas* similar to *Pseudomonas marginatia* are responsible for most soft rot of onions during transportation or in storage. These micro-organisms develop on onions in the field before harvesting after heavily rains and when leaves are drying. The main source of inoculums is contaminated soil and crop Residues. The bacteria are spread by splashing rain, irrigation water, and insects. Which enter into the bulbs only through wounds such as those cause by transplanting, mechanical injuries or sunscald, it is said that the spoilage of onions occur during storage because *Pseudomonas aeroginosa* contaminates onion bulbs during harvest by moving through wounds caused by topping, finally causing soft rot. The pathogen can also be seed borne. Botrytis neck rot is caused by a different pathogen from Botrytis leaf spot. This is seen primarily in onion, the spoilage occur more apparently after harvest, while bulbs are in storage. At first the soft neck tissues looks water soaked, and a yellow discoloration moves down into the scales. Bulbs break down into soft mass. A gray mold develops between the onion scales, later producing small to large black bodies (sclerotia) which develop as solid layer around the neck (Carisse *et al.*, 2015).

Spoilage microorganism can also cause spoilage by entering plant tissue during development either through the calyx along the stem, or through various specialized water and gas exchange structures of leafy matter. Blue mold of onion spoilage this is caused by several *Penicillium* species. These fungi, attack a wide range of vegetables, bulbs, and seeds they are common in the soil growing in infected animal and plant debris. These organisms develop on lesions when bulbs are cut open, one or more of the fleshy scales may be discolored and water soaked. These microorganisms are responsible for poor plant stand in the field and storage delay. The presence of fungi in onions bulbs is also attributed to the environmental conditions, state of handling and processing, state of storage facility and the onions the fungal load of the handlers and the quality of the onion bulbs. These fungi have been known to cause disease of humans and animals.

2.4 Antioxidant effects of *A. cepa*

Oxidative stress is characterised by over production of reactive oxygen species (ROS) and reactive nitrogen species (RNS) (Abdel-salam *et al*. 2014). These free radicals, mainly nitric oxide, superoxide anion, hydroxyl radical and hydrogen peroxide, can cause oxidative damages to nucleic acids, proteins, and lipids. Thus, excess production of free radicals under pro-inflammatory conditions may initiate various diseases (Alpsoy *et al*., 2013). Natural antioxidants are compounds that can delay or inhibit oxidative reactions by scavenging free radicals. The most important of these compounds are phenolic acids, polyphenols, flavonoids, alkaloids and terpenoids (Brewster, 2018). Therefore, suppression of oxidative stress could be achieved by using potential sources of natural antioxidants such as medicinal plants (Celik, 2012). Essential oils derived from these plants, are rich sources of antioxidant components with different biological activities (Colina-Coca *et al*., 2017). *A. cepa* contains high levels of phenolic compounds mainly flavonoids, which have antioxidant properties besides other pharmacological effects such as antibiotic, antidiabetic, anti-atherogenic and anticancer activities (Liguori *et al*. 2017). Flavones, flavanones, flavonols, isoflavones, flavanonols, chalcones, and anthocyanins which are subclasses of flavonoids and flavonols, are the most abundant flavonoids in *A. cepa* (Liguori *et al*. 2017). Several studies reported the antioxidant activities of *A. cepa* and its constituents and introduced the plant as a potential source of natural antioxidants (Razavi *et al*., 2016). Alterations in oxidant/antioxidant markers including lipid peroxidation (LPO), glutathione (GSH), superoxide dismutase (SOD), catalase (CAT), and MDA were observed by studies that investigated the effects of *A. cepa* and its constituents (Liguori *et al.*, 2017).

2.5 Antimicrobial activity

Allium cepa has been described as a potent antimicrobial agent to fight against infectious diseases. Many bacteria, fungi, and viruses were found to be susceptible to different solvents extracts of *A. cepa*. Sulphur compounds have proven to be the principal active antimicrobial agent present in onion (Rose *et al.* 2015). Many studies (Liguori *et al.* 2017; Thomas and Parkin, 2010; Vazquez-Armenta *et al.*, 2014) have reconsidered the effect of organo-sulphur containing compounds on the growth of microorganisms. *A. cepa* also possesses other antimicrobial phenolic compounds including protocatechuic, p-coumaric, ferulic acids, and catechol. Quercetin and kaempferol have been found as significant contributors to this activity. The effectiveness of kaempferol was greater than quercetin in inhibiting bacterial growth of *B. cereus*, *L. monocytogenes*, and *P. aeruginosa* and was as effective as quercetin in inhibiting the growth of *S. aureus* and *M. luteus* (Santas *et al.* (2010). Other studies also showed that quercetin oxidation products from yellow onion skin such as 2-(3,4-dihydroxyphenyl)-4,6-dihydroxy2-methoxybenzofuran-3-one demonstrated selective activity against *Helicobacter pylori* strains while 3-(quercetin-8-yl)- 2,3-epoxyflavanone showed antibacterial activity against both multi-drug resistant *Staphylococcus aureus* and *H. pylori* strains (Ramos *et al.* 2016). Benkeblia (2014) observed that essential oil of three types of onion (yellow, green and, red) displayed marked antimicrobial activity against specific pathogens, including *Staphylococcus aureus*, *Salmonella enteritidis*, *Aspergillus niger*, *Penicillium cyclopium*, and *Fusarium oxysporum* (Benkeblia 2014). Several researchers such as Begum and Yassen 2015;

12

Hamza 2015; Palaksha *et al.* 2013 and Zohri *et al.* (2010) have studied the activity of onion extracts on the Gram-negative bacteria *Klebsiella* spp. However, contradicting results were obtained from Srinivasan *et al.* (2011) and Gomaa (2017) whereby there was no inhibition of *K. pneumonia* with onion extracts. The antibacterial activity of the red variety of *A. cepa* extract was found to be higher compared to yellow and white varieties (Sharma *et al.* 2017). Interestingly, Azu *et al.* (2017) found that *A. cepa* was effective against *P. aeruginosa* isolated from patients suffering from urinary tract infections indicating its potential in the management of such condition. In vivo study of Ur Rahman *et al.* (2017) showed that birds fed with onion at a rate of 2.5 g/kg of feed had a decrease of *E. coli* population and a significant increase of *Lactobacillus* spp. Interestingly, a recent study conducted by Lekshmi *et al.* (2012) showed how nanoparticles synthesized from onion displayed a positive effect in inhibiting *Klebsiella* spp. Saxena *et al.* (2010) also reported the synthesis of silver nanoparticles by using onion extract and demonstrated that these nanoparticles, at a concentration of 50 lg/mL, presented a complete antibacterial activity against *E. coli* and *Salmonella typhimurium*. Onion extracts are potent against fungal species, and its essential oil inhibits the dermatophyte fungi (Zohri *et al.* 2010). *Aspergillus niger* and *Fusarium oxysporum* were strongly inhibited (minimum fungicidal concentration (MFC) ¼ 75 and 100 mg/mL, respectively) by the ethyl alcohol extract of dehydrated onion (Irkin and Korukluoglu 2017; Irkin and Korukluoglu 2019). Anti-fungal saponins (ceposide A and C) discovered by Lanzotti *et al.* (2012) were able to inhibit the growth of soil-borne pathogens (R. solani), air-borne pathogens (*A. alternata, B. cenerea, Mucor* spp and *Phomopsis* spp) and antagonistic fungi (*T. atroviride* and *T. harzianum*). High inhibitory effect against *M. furfur* (minimum inhibitory concentration (MIC) ¼ 8.062 mg/ml) and *C. albicans* (MIC ¼4.522 mg/ml) were reported by Shams-Ghahfarokhi *et al.*

13

(2016). Kocic-Tanackov *et al.* (2019) stated that essential oil of *A. cepa*, at a concentration of 7%, had complete inhibition on the growth of two yeasts (*C. tropicalis* and *S. cerevisiae*) and this was also confirmed by the study of Kivanc and Kunduhoglu (2010). High concentration of the essential oil also weakened the growth of molds (*A. tamarii* and *P. griseofulvum*) as well and complete inhibition was observed for *E. astelodami*. Goren *et al.* (2012) conducted a clinical experiment to find out if dehydrated *A. cepa* could be used in the treatment of AIDS. Eight persons (from 28 to 30 years old) who were HIV positive started a dietary regimen comprising of 9–13 g/day of *A. cepa* extract. After the treatment, all the HIV positive patients experienced a total remission of clinical symptoms associated with AIDS and were able to resume their healthy lifestyle.

3.0 MATERIALS AND METHODS

3.1 Study Area

The study was conducted during the months of October to December, 2021 in the Microbiology Laboratory, University of Abuja in Gwagwalada Area Council, in the Federal Capital Territory, Abuja, Nigeria. It is located geographically at the North Central part of Nigeria between latitude 8.941° and longitude 7.092°, with a population of 158,618 people (National Population Commission Nigeria, 2006). The temperature of the area ranges from 30–37°C yearly with the highest temperature experienced in the month of March and with mean total rainfall approximately 1,650 mm per annum. The area as a whole is located within the northern boundary of the guinea savannah. The rainy season begins from April and ends in October, while day time temperature reaches 28 °C to 30°C and night time temperature of 22°C to 23°C. The rainy season is from March to November with a mean annual rainfall of about 1400 mm.

3.2 Materials used and Sterilization

The sterilization of glass wares such as conical flasks, beaker and test tubes after washing with detergent was carried out in hot air oven at 160 °C for 2 hours.

3.3 Collection of Samples

Healthy onion bulbs were collected randomly from two selected markets in Gwagwalada: Kaswandare market and Gwagwalada main market and then brought to the Microbiology laboratory, to evaluate the effect of fungal infestation on the antioxidant properties of onion bulbs stored in sack.

3.4   Storage of Onion Bulb in Sack Bag

Onion bulb showing symptoms of rotting and discolouration were sorted out and the healthy ones were selected. The healthy selected onion from the two locations was separately stored in two different sack bags and then stored at ambient temperature for 14 days. The fungal infestation and antioxidant properties of the onion bulbs stored in the sack bags was then be analysed at day zero (0), day 7 and day 14 respectively.

3.5   Preparation and sterilization of media

Potato dextrose agar (PDA) was use in this study and prepared according to the manufacturer's instructions thus, 39g of the PDA was dissolved in 1000ml of sterile water and then sterilized (autoclaved) at 121°C and pressure of 15Pa for 15 minutes. Potato dextrose agar was use for the isolation of infested fungi and maintenance of pure cultures of the isolated fungi.

3.6   Assessment of Fungal Infestation of the Onion bulb during Storage

Fungal infestation of the onion bulb during storage was assessed using the blotter method as described by Dimka and Onuegbu (2010). The Onion bulb surface was disinfected using 2% hypochlorite and then rinsed three (3) times with distilled water. About 1 gram of disinfected onion bulb was aseptically placed on already prepared Potato dextrose agar plates. The inoculated plates were incubated at ambient temperature ($25 \pm 2\ ^0C$) for 5 days.

3.6.1 Preparation of pure cultures of fungal isolates

The young fungal colonies were aseptically picked up and transferred to fresh sterile PDA plates to obtain pure cultures.

3.7 Identification of fungal isolates

Isolates obtained were characterized and identified on the basis of their colonial and morphological characteristics which include macroscopic and microscopic examinations. Among the characteristics to be use are colonial characteristics such as size, surface appearance, texture and pigmentation of the colonies (Sharma and Rajak 2003). In addition, microscopy revealed vegetative mycelium including presence or absence of cross-walls, diameter of hyphae, and types of asexual and sexual reproductive structures. Slide culture method that minimized serious distortion of sporing structures was used. Appropriate references were then made using mycological identification keys and taxonomic description.

3.8 Determination of Frequency of Occurrence of Fungal Isolates

The frequency of occurrence was determined by taking the sum of all the numbers of fungal in each sample and the percentage was calculated as:

$$\frac{\text{Number of each Isolates} \times 100}{\text{Total number of Isolates}}$$

3.9 Preparation of Onion Extract

Aqueous extract of the fungal infested and un-infested (control) Onion bulb was prepared separately. About 100gm of the onion bulb was blended using electric blender then transfer into 1000ml Erlermeyer flask and 500ml of the distilled water was added into each container. The content was mixed and kept in bioshaker for 24 hours. After 24 hours, the content in the flask was filtered using Whattman no.1 filter paper and then concentrated by evaporation, using water bath.

3.10   Determination of antioxidant Properties of Onion

3.10.1   DPPH Free radical scavenging assay

The antioxidant capacity of the Onion was evaluated by the free radical scavenging and the effect on the 1,1- diphenyl- 2- picrylhydrazyl (DPPH) radical. The determination was assessed by using procedure reported by Sultana *et al.* (2018). Briefly, 5.0ml of a freshly prepared solution of 1, 1- diphenyl- 2- picryhydrazyl (DPPH) ethanolic solution at concentration of 0.025g/l was added to 1.0ml of extract containing 25g/ml of dry matter in ethanol. The mixture was shake and kept in the dark and left to stand at room temperature for 30 mins. The absorbance of the resulting solution was measured at 515nm, against a blank of ethanol without DPPH, using a UV-visible spectrophotometer (Shimadzu UV- 1601PC, Tokyo, Japan). Results were expressed as percentage (%) of inhibition of the DPPH radical which was calculated according to the following equation; % DPPH = (Abs control- Abs sample)/(Abs control) x 100. Where Abs control is the absorbance of DPPH solution without extracts

3.10.2 Measurement of reducing power of the crude extracts of Onion Bulb

Reducing power of the crude extracts of spices was determined according to the method of Sultana *et al.* (2018). The crude extract (5ml) of Onion (5 ml) was mixed with equal volume of 0.2 M phosphate buffer (pH, 6.6) and 1 % potassium ferricyanide. The mixture was incubated at 50 °C for 20 min, after which an equal volume of 1 % trichloro acetic acid (TCA) was added to the mixture and then centrifuged at 3000 rpm for 10 min. The upper layer (the supernatant) of the suspension was mixed with distilled water and 0.1 % $FeCl_3$ in the ratio of 1:1:2, and the absorbance measured at 700 nm. Increased absorbance of the reaction mixture indicated increased reducing power.

3.10.3 Determination of antioxidant activity of crude extracts of the Onion

The ferric thiocyanate (FTC) method was adopted from Sultana *et al*. (2008) method. The crude extracts o the onion bulb (2.5 ml) was separately added to 2.5 ml of 95% (V/V) ethanol, and then mixed with 4.1 ml of linoleic acid (2.51 % V/V) in 99.5 % (V/V) ethanol, 8ml of 0.05 M phosphate buffer (pH 7.0), 3.9 ml of distilled water and then kept in the dark in screw- capped containers at 4 $^{\circ}$C. To 0.1 ml of this solution, 9.7 ml of 75 % (V/V) ethanol and 0.1 ml of 30 % (W/V) ammonium thiocyanate was added. A 0.1 ml volume of 20 mM Ferrous chloride in 3.5 % (V/V) hydrochloric acid was added to the reaction mixture, and the absorbance of the resulting red solution measured after 3 min at 500 nm repeatedly at interval of 24 h until the control (no extract) reached the maximum value. This was carried out in duplicates and results averaged. The percentage inhibition of linoleic acid peroxidation was calculated as:

$$(\%) \text{ Inhibition} = 100 - \left\{ \frac{(\text{Absorbance increase of sample X 100})}{(\text{Absorbance increase of blank})} \right\}$$

3.11 Statistical Analysis
The statistical analysis was determined using one way Analysis of Variance (ANOVA) from Ms Excel Statistics. Test applied was F-test statistic at p= 0.05.

4.0 RESULTS

4.1 Fungal Infestation of Onion Bulbs during Storage in Sack

Table 1 shows the fungal infestation of onion bulbs during storage in sack. The fungal infestation of onion bulbs during storage in sack as seen in Table 1 shows that five (5) fungi each were isolated from the onion bulbs during storage in sack at day zero (0) and day seven (7) respectively while at day fourteen (14), six fungal infestation was isolated from the onion bulbs during storage in sack as seen in Table 1.

Table 1: Fungal Infestation of Onion Bulbs during Storage in Sack

Duration of Storage	Number of Sample	Isolates	Frequency	
		Aspergillus fumigatus	2	
Day Zero (0)	5	*Aspergillus flavus*	2	
		Rhizopus stolonifer	1	
		Total		**5**
		Aspergillus niger		3
Day Seven (7)	5	*Aspergillus flavus*	1	
		Fusarium oxysporum	1	
		Total		**5**
		Aspergillus niger		2
		Penicillium chrysogenum		1
Day Fourteen (14)	5	*Aspergillus flavus*	2	
		Fusarium oxysporum	1	
		Total		**6**
Overall Total	**15**		**16**	

20

4.2 Frequency and Percentages of Fungal Infestation of Onion Bulbs

Table 2 shows that a total of sixteen (16) fungi infested the onion bulbs during storage in sack.

The fungi belong to four (5) genera and six (6) species of fungi infested the onion bulbs during

storage in sack. *Aspersillus niger* and *Aspersillus flavus* were the most frequently isolated fungi

with 31.25% each followed by *Fusarium oxysporum* and *Aspergillus fumigatus* with 12.50% each

while *Penicillium chrysogenum* and *Rhizopus stolonifer* recorded 6.25% each as seen in Table 2.

Table 2: Frequency and Percentage of Fungal Infestation of Onion Bulbs during Storage in Sack

Fungi Isolates	Frequencies of Occurrence	Percentages (%)
Aspersillus niger	5	31.25
Aspergillus flavus	5	31.25
Aspergillus fumigatus	2	12.50
Fusarium oxysporum	2	12.50
Penicillium chrysogenum	1	6.25
Rhizopus stolonifer	1	6.25
Total	**16**	**100**

4.3   DPPH radical scavenging activity of Fungal Infested Onion Bulbs
during Storage in Sack

The antioxidant analysis of onion extract after storage in sack for 14 days is represented in Table

3 respectively. At all concentrations (0.5, 0.25, 0.125, 0.0625 and 0.03125 mg/ml), the antioxidant

property of the onion extract at day zero (0) and day 7 was higher than that 14. The inhibition of

free radical DPPH at day zero (0) and 7 were 29.92 %, 49.21%, 69.29%, 70.07% and 47.63% while

at day 14, the percentage (%) of inhibition of free radical DPPH were 29.33 %, 49.02%, 69.01%,

69.77% and 47.21% as seen in Table 3.

Table 3: Antioxidant analysis of Onion Extract after storage in Sack for 14 days

Concentration (mg/ml)	% inhibition of Vitamin C	% inhibition of Onion Extracts		
		Day 0	Day 7	Day 14
0.5	70.07	29.92	29.92	29.33
0.25	72.83	49.21	49.21	49.02
0.125	75.59	69.29	69.29	69.01
0.0625	75.19	70.07	70.07	69.77
0.03125	74.80	47.63	47.63	47.21

5.0 DISCUSSIONS AND CONCLUSION

5.1 Discussions

It appears from this study that the fungal infestation of onion bulbs during storage in sack shows that five (5) fungi each were isolated from the onion bulbs during storage in sack at day zero (0) and day seven (7) respectively while at day fourteen (14), six fungal infestation was isolated from the onion bulbs during storage in sack. Under conditions of rapid movement of bulbs from field to market, it is likely that the effects of the other fungi may be negligible. However, onions are frequently stored for 1-5 months after harvest in Nigeria. Visser (2019) published that injury to the bulb incurred during storage and this was the key factor in storage disease development causing storage loss. The results of this present study indicate that the fungal infestations in storage of onion are higher in onions stored in sack.

The finding from this study indicates that a total of sixteen (16) fungi infested the onion bulbs during storage in sack. The fungi belong to four (5) genera and six (6) species of fungi infested the onion bulbs during storage in sack. *Aspersillus niger* and *Aspersillus flavus* were the most frequently isolated fungi with 31.25% each followed by *Fusarium oxysporum* and *Aspergillus fumigatus* with 12.50% each while *Penicillium chrysogenum* and *Rhizopus stolonifer* recorded 6.25% each.

This agrees with the reports of other researchers (Muhammad *et al.*, 2004; Dimka and Onuegbu, 2010) that fungi constitute a menace in the storage of many agricultural commodities including fruits, vegetables and nuts. Latent infection of onion bulbs may be the main factor contributing to postharvest deterioration during storage. Microbial infection of bulbs is often the result of poor preharvest management practices. A certain level of postharvest rots of onion bulbs is inevitable, because their perishable nature, but this should be kept to a minimum.

Srinivasan and Shanmugam (2016) evaluated the efficacy of six types of containers/methods viz., jute gunny bags, polythene lined gunny bag with perforations, bamboo basket, bamboo bins, wooden rake and hanging method in reducing the spoilage in stored onions. They reported that containers used for storage of onion bulbs showed significant influence on the incidence and development of *Aspergillus niger* rot.

The results revealed that onion extract has a great antioxidant capacity and exhibited a significant relation between phenolic content and antioxidant activity of the plant. At all concentrations (0.5, 0.25, 0.125, 0.0625 and 0.03125 mg/ml), the antioxidant property of the onion extract at day zero (0) and day 7 was higher than that 14. The inhibition of free radical DPPH at day zero (0) and 7 were 29.92 %, 49.21%, 69.29%, 70.07% and 47.63% while at day 14, the percentage (%) of inhibition of free radical DPPH were 29.33 %, 49.02%, 69.01%, 69.77% and 47.21%. Similarly, Joung and Jung (2014) also reported that the antioxidant activity of onion peels extracts was assessed by DPPH radical scavenging activity. The results suggested that onion extracts have a remarkable antioxidant activity.

The radical scavenging and antioxidant activities of extracts of of *A. cepa*, were also investigated by Škerget *et al.* (2009) and the results showed a robust radical scavenging potential for the onion extract. This agrees with the finding of this study.

5.2   Conclusion

It can be concluded from this study that *Aspersillus niger, Aspersillus flavus, Fusarium oxysporum, Aspergillus fumigates, Penicillium chrysogenum* and *Rhizopus stolonifer* were the common fungi that infested onion bulbs during storage in sack. Also, it appears that the effects of the fungi infestation on the antioxidant activity of the onion bulbs were not significantly high.

5.3   Recommendation

Healthy, undamaged onion bulbs which have been dried in the field should be stored in dry well-ventilated stores. This will reduce growth and development of fungal pathogens and minimize storage rots.

Therefore, *A. cepa* and its constituents could be of therapeutic value in disorders such as aging, anti-inflammatory, and wound healing processes where radical scavenging activity can be of therapeutic value.

REFERENCES

Abdel-Salam, A., Shahenda, M., E. and Jehan, B., A. (2014). Antimicrobial and antioxidant activities of red onion, garlic and leek in sausage. *African Journal of Microbiology Research*, 8 (27):2574–82.

Adamick, I.F. (2014). Effects of pre-harvest treatments and storage conditions on quality and shelf-life of onions. *Acta Horticulture (ISHS), 688: 229-238.*

Adebayo, L. O. and Diyaolu, S. A. (2013). Mycology and spoilage of cashew nuts. *African Journal of Biotechnology*, 2: 369-373

Akash, M. S. H., Rehman, K. and Chen, S. (2014). Spice plant *Allium cepa*: Dietary supplement for treatment of type 2 diabetes mellitus. *Nutrition*, 30 (10):1128–37.

Al-Hindi, R.R., Al-Najada, A.R. and Mohammed, S.A. (2011). Isolation and identification of some fruit spoilage fungi: screening of plant cell wall degrading enzymes. *African Journal of microbiology Research, 5 (4): 443-448.*

Alpsoy, S., Aktas, C., Uygur, R., Topcu, B., Kanter, M., Erboga, M., Karakaya, O. and Gedikbasi, A. (2013). Antioxidant and anti-apoptotic effects of onion (*Allium cepa*) extract on doxorubicin-induced cardiotoxicity in rats. *Journal of Applied Toxicology*, 33 (3):202–8.

Azu, N. C., Onyeagba, R. A., Nworie, O. and Kalu, J. (2017). Antibacterial activity of *Allium cepa* (onions) and *Zingiber officinale* (ginger) on *Staphylococcus aureus* and *Pseudomonas aeruginosa* isolated from high vaginal swab. *The Internet Journal of Tropical Medicine*, 3 (2):1540–2681.

Begum, H. A., and Yassen, T. (2015). Anitmicrobial, phytochemical, ethnobotanical and proximate analysis of *Allium cepa* L. *Journal of Advanced Botany and Zoology*, 3 (1):1–4.

Benkeblia, N. (2014). Antimicrobial activity of essential oil extracts of various onions (Allium cepa) and garlic (*Allium sativum*). *Food Science and Technology*, 37 (2):263–8.

Brewster, J. L. (2018). Onions and other vegetable alliums. UK: Biddles Ltd. Campos, K., Y. Diniz, A. Cataneo, L. Faine, M. Alves, and E. Novelli. 2013. Hypoglycaemic and antioxidant effects of onion, *Allium cepa*: dietary onion addition, antioxidant activity and hypoglycaemic effects on diabetic rats. *International Journal of Food Sciences and Nutrition*, 54 (3):241–6.

Carisse, O., Tremblay, D.M, Brodeur, L., Mc Donald, M.R. and Mc Roberts, N. (2015). Management of Botrytis leaf blight of onion. *The quebea experience of 20 years of continual improvement plant disease, 95: 504-514.*

Celik, T. A. (2012). Potential genotoxic and cytotoxic effects of plant extracts. In A Compendium of Essays on Alternative Therapy, ed. Bhattacharya A. InTech. Che Othman, S. F., S. O. Idid, S. Z. Idid, M. S. Koya, A. Mohamed Rehan, and K. R. Kamarudin. Antioxidant study of garlic and red onion: a comparative study. *Pertanika Journal of Tropical Agricultural Science*, 34:253–61.

Colina-Coca, C., Gonz_alez-Pe~na, D., de Ancos, B. and Sanchez- Moreno, C. (2017). Dietary onion ameliorates antioxidant defence, inflammatory response, and cardiovascular risk biomarkers in hypercholesterolemic wistar rats. *Journal of Functional Foods*, 36:300–9.

Corzo-Martınez, M., Corzo, N. and Villamiel, M. (2017). Biological properties of onions and garlic. *Trends in Food Science and Technology*, 18 (12):609–25.

Dimka, S. O. N. and Onuegbu, B. A. (2010). Mycoflora of copra and effect of brining on some properties of copra in Nigeria. *Agriculture and Biology Journal of North America*, 111: 2151 – 7525

Dimka, S. O. N. and Onuegbu, B. A. (2010). Mycoflora of copra and effect of brining on some properties of copra in Nigeria. *Agriculture and Biology Journal of North America*, 111: 2151 – 7525

Dogondaji, S.D.., Baba, K.M., Muhammad, I. and Magaji, M.D. (2015). Evaluation of onion storage losses and implication for food security in Sokoto Metropolis. *Bulletin of Science Association of Nigeria*, 26: 10 – 14.

Dogondaji, S.D.., Baba, K.M., Muhammad, I. and Magaji, M.D. (2015). Evaluation of onion storage losses and implication for food security in Sokoto Metropolis. *Bulletin of Science Association of Nigeria*, 26: 10 – 14.

Ferreres, F., Gil, M. I. and Tomas-Barberan, F. A. (2010). Anthocyanins and flavonoids from shredded red onion and changes during storage in perforated films. *Food Research International*, 29 (3–4):389–95.

Fossen, T., Pedersen, A.T. and Andersen, O.M. (2011). Flavonoids from red onion (Allium cepa). *Phytochemistry*, 47(2):281–285.

Fossen, T., Pedersen, A.T. and Andersen, O.M. (2011). Flavonoids from red onion (Allium cepa). *Phytochemistry*, 47(2):281–285.

Gashua, I.B. Ukekpe, U.S. and Abba, A.M. (2014). Refractometric analysis of some local onion cultivars (*Allium Cepa* L) Bulbs for dehydration. *European Journal of Applied science, 6(1), 07-10.*

Gent, D.H. and Mohan, S.K. (2016). Iris yellow spot virus an emerging threat to onion bulb and seed production. *Plant disease, 90: 1468-1480.*

Gomaa, E. Z. (2017). Antimicrobial, antioxidant and antitumor activities of silver nanoparticles synthesized by *Allium cepa* extract: A green approach. *Journal of Genetic Engineering and Biotechnology,* 15(1):49–57.

Goren, A., Goldman, W. F., Trainin, Z. and Goldman, S. R. (2012). Antiviral composition derived from *Allium cepa* and therapeutic use thereof. *Journal of Agricultural and Food Chemistry,* 56 (12):4418–26.

Gupta, R., Thakur, B., Singh, P., Singh, H., Sharma, V., Katoch, V. and Chauhan, S.(2010). Anti-tuberculosis activity of selected medicinal plants against multi-drug resistant *Mycobacterium tuberculosis* isolates. *Indian Journal of Medical Research,* 131:809–13.

Hamza, H. (2015). Antimicrobial activity of some plant extracts on microbial pathogens isolated from Hilla city hospitals. *Iraq Medical Journal Babylon,* 12:398–407.

Hayta, S., Polat, R, and Selvi, S. (2014). Traditional uses of medicinal plants in Elazı_g (Turkey). *Journal of Ethnopharmacology,* 154 (3):613–23.

Ioku, K., Aoyama, Y. and Tokuno, A. (2011). Various cooking methods and the flavonoid content in onion. *Journal of Nutritional Science and Vitaminology,* 47(1): 78–83.

Ioku, K., Aoyama, Y. and Tokuno, A. (2011). Various cooking methods and the flavonoid content in onion. *Journal of Nutritional Science and Vitaminology,* 47(1): 78–83.

Irkin, R. and K orukluoglu, M. (2017). Control of Aspergillus niger with garlic, onion and leek extracts. *African Journal of Biotechnology,* 6:384–387

Irkin, R., and Korukluoglu, M. (2019). Control of some filamentous fungi and yeasts by dehydrated allium extracts. *Journal F€ur Verbraucherschutz Und Lebensmittelsicherheit,* 4 (1):3–6.

Jaradat, N. A., Ayesh, O. I. and Anderson, C. (2016). Ethnopharmacological survey about medicinal plants utilized by herbalists and traditional practitioner healers for treatments of diarrhea in the West Bank/Palestine. *Journal of Ethnopharmacology,* 182:57–66.

Joung EM, Jung KH.. 2014. Antioxidant activity of onion (*Allium cepa* L.) peel extracts obtained as onion byproducts. *Korean Journal of Food Science Technology,* 46(3): 364–368

Kabrah, A. (2010). The antibacterial activity of onion on MSSA and MRSA isolates of *Staphylococcus aureus. Biomedical Sciences,* 1:24–64.

Kivanc, M. and Kunduhoglu, B. (2010). Antimicrobial activity of fresh plant juice on the growth of bacteria and yeasts. *Journal of Qafqaz University*, 1:27–35.

Kocic-Tanackov, S. D., Dimic, G. P., Tepic, A. C. and Vujicic, B. L. (2019). Influence of *allium ampeloprasum* L. and *allium cepa* L. essential oils on the growth of some yeasts and moulds. *Zbornik Matice Srpske Za Prirodne Nauke*, 116:121–30.

Krest, I. and Keusgen, M. (2012). Biosensoric flowthrough method for the determination of cysteine sulfoxides. *Analytical Chemistry Journal*, 469(2): 155–164.

Krest, I. and Keusgen, M. (2012). Biosensoric flowthrough method for the determination of cysteine sulfoxides. *Analytical Chemistry Journal*, 469(2): 155–164.

Lanzotti, V., Romano, A., Lanzuise, S., Bonanomi, G. and Scala, F. (2012). Antifungal saponins from bulbs of white onion, *Allium cepa* L. *Phytochemistry*, 74:133–9.

Lekshmi, N. P., Sumi, S. B., Viveka, S., Jeeva, S. and Brindha, J. R. (2012). Antibacterial activity of nanoparticles from *allium* sp. *Journal of Microbiology and Biotechnology Research*, 2:115–9.

Liguori, L., Califano, R., Albanese, D., Raimo, F., Crescitelli, A, and Di Matteo, M. (2017). Chemical composition and antioxidant properties of five white onion (*Allium cepa* L.) landraces. *Journal of Food Quality*, 2017:1–9.

Muhammad, S. Shehu, K. and Amusa, N. A. (2014). Survey of the market Diseases and aflatoxin contamination of tomato (*Lycopersiconescolentus*Mill.)Fruits in Sokoto, Northwestern Nigeria. *Nutrition and food science*, 34 (2): 72-76

Muhammad, S. Shehu, K. and Amusa, N. A. (2014). Survey of the market Diseases and aflatoxin contamination of tomato (*Lycopersiconescolentus*Mill.)Fruits in Sokoto, Northwestern Nigeria. *Nutrition and food science*, 34 (2): 72-76

Narayana, K.J.P., Srikanth, M. and Vijayalakshmi, M. (2017). Toxic spectrum of aspergilus Niger causing black mold rot of onions. *Research Journal of Microbiology*, 2(11): 881–884

Ole, H., Torben, L., Lars, P.C., Ulla, K., Nazmul, H. and Shakuntala H.A. (2014). Contents of Iron Zinc, and β - ca-rotene in Commonly consumed vegetables in Bangla-desh. *Journal of Food Composition and Analysis*, 17: 587–595.

Ole, H., Torben, L., Lars, P.C., Ulla, K., Nazmul, H. and Shakuntala H.A. (2014). Contents of Iron Zinc, and β - ca-rotene in Commonly consumed vegetables in Bangla-desh. *Journal of Food Composition and Analysis*, 17: 587–595.

Palaksha, M., Banji, D. and Rao, A. (2013). In-vitro evaluation of antibacterial activity of alcoholic extracts of ten South Indian spices against multi-resistant gram positive and gram negative bacteria by agar well diffusion method. *World Journal of Pharmacy and Pharmaceutical Sciences*, 2:3840–7.

Ramos, F. A., Takaishi, Y., Shirotori, M., Kawaguchi, Y., Tsuchiya, K., Shibata, H., Higuti, T., Tadokoro, T. and Takeuchi, M. (2016). Antibacterial and antioxidant activities of quercetin oxidation products from yellow onion (*Allium cepa*) skin. *Journal of Agricultural and Food Chemistry*, 54 (10):3551–7.

Razavi-Azarkhiavi, K., Behravan, J., Mosaffa, F., Sehatbakhsh, S., Shirani, K. and Karimi, G. (2014). Protective effects of aqueous and ethanol extracts of rosemary on H_2O_2-induced oxidative DNA damage in human lymphocytes by comet assay. *Journal of Complementary and Integrative Medicine*, 11:27–33.

Rose, P., Whiteman, M., Moore, P. K. and Zhu, Y. Z. (2015). Bioactive Salk (en) yl cysteine sulfoxide metabolites in the genus allium: the chemistry of potential therapeutic agents. *Natural Product Reports*, 36 (35):351–68.

Samuel, O. and Ifeanyi, O. (2015). Fungi associated with the deterioration of post harvest onion bulb sold in some markets in Awka, Nigeria. *Journal of Bioengineering and Bioscience,* 3(5): 90–94.

Santas, J., Almajano, M. P. and Carbo, R. (2010). Antimicrobial and antioxidant activity of crude onion (*Allium cepa*, L.) extracts. *International Journal of Food Science and Technology*, 45 (2):403–9.

Saxena, A., Tripathi, R. and Singh, R. (2010). Biological synthesis of silver nanoparticles by using onion (*Allium cepa*) extract and their antibacterial activity. *Digest Journal of Nanomaterials and Biostructures*, 5:427–32.

Shams-Ghahfarokhi, M., Shokoohamiri, M. R., Amirrajab, N., Moghadasi, B., Ghajari, A., Zeini, F., Sadeghi, G. and Razzaghi- Abyaneh, M. (2016). In vitro antifungal activities of *Allium cepa, allium sativum* and ketoconazole against some pathogenic yeasts and dermatophytes. *Fitoterapia*, 77(4):321–3.

Sharma, J., Gairola, S., Sharma, Y, P. and Gaur, R. (2014). Ethnomedicinal plants used to treat skin diseases by tharu community of district Udham Singh Nagar, Uttarakhand, India. *Journal of Ehnopharmacology*, 158 :140–206.

Sharma, K., Mahato, N. and Lee, Y. R. (2017). Systematic study on active compounds as antibacterial and antibiofilm agent in aging onions. *Journal of food and drug analysis,* 26:518–28.

Shehu, K. and Muhammad, S. (2011). Fungi associated with the storage rots of onion bulb in Sokoto Nigeria. *International journal of modern Botany*, 1(1):1–3.

Silambarasan, R. and Ayyanar, M. (2015). An ethnobotanical study of medicinal plants in palamalai region of Eastern ghats, India. *Journal of Ehnopharmacology*, 172:162–78.

Škerget M, Majhenič L, Bezjak M, Knez Ž.. 2009. Antioxidant, radical scavenging and antimicrobial activities of red onion (*Allium cepa* L) skin and edible part extracts. *Chemistry, Biochemistry and Engineering*, 23:435–444

Srinivasan, D., Nathan, S., Suresh, T. and Perumalsamy, P. L. (2011). Antimicrobial activity of certain indian medicinal plants used in folkloric medicine. *Journal of Ethnopharmacology*, 74(3):217–20.

Srinivasan, R. and Shanmugam, V. (2016). Post harvest management of black mould rot of onion. *IndianPhytopathology*, 59 (3): 333-339

Sultana, B., Anwar, F., Asi, M.R and Chatha, S.A.S. (2008). Antioxidant potential of extracts from different agro wastes. *Stailization of corn oil*, *Grasasy Aceites*, 59(3): 205- 217.

Sultana, B., Anwar, F., Asi, M.R and Chatha, S.A.S. (2018). Antioxidant potential of extracts from different agro wastes. *Stailization of corn oil*, *Grasasy Aceites*, 59(3): 205- 217.

Thomas, D. J. and Parkin, K. L. (2010). Quantification of alk (en) yl- L-cysteine sulfoxides and related amino acids in alliums by highperformance liquid chromatography. *Journal of Agricultural and Food Chemistry*, 42(8):1632–8.

Ur Rahman, S., Khan, S., Chand, N., Sadique, U. and Khan, R. U. (2017). In vivo effects of *Allium cepa* L. on the selected gut microflora and intestinal histomorphology in broiler. *Acta Histochemica*, 119 (5):446–50.

Vazquez-Armenta, F., Ayala-Zavala, J., Olivas, G., Molina-Corral, F. and Silva-Espinoza, B. (2014). Antibrowning and antimicrobial effects of onion essential oil to preserve the quality of cut potatoes. *Acta Alimentaria*, 43(4):640–9.

Visser, C.L.M. (2019). *Fusarium* in onions and varietal differences in infection: evaluation of a biotest. *PAV Bulletin Vollegronds groenteteelt*. 4-7.

Zohri, A.N., Abdel-Gawad, K. and Saber, S. (2010). Antibacterial, antidermatophytic and antitoxigenic activities of onion (*Allium cepa* L.) oil. *Microbiological Research*, 150 (2):167–72.

YOUR KNOWLEDGE HAS VALUE

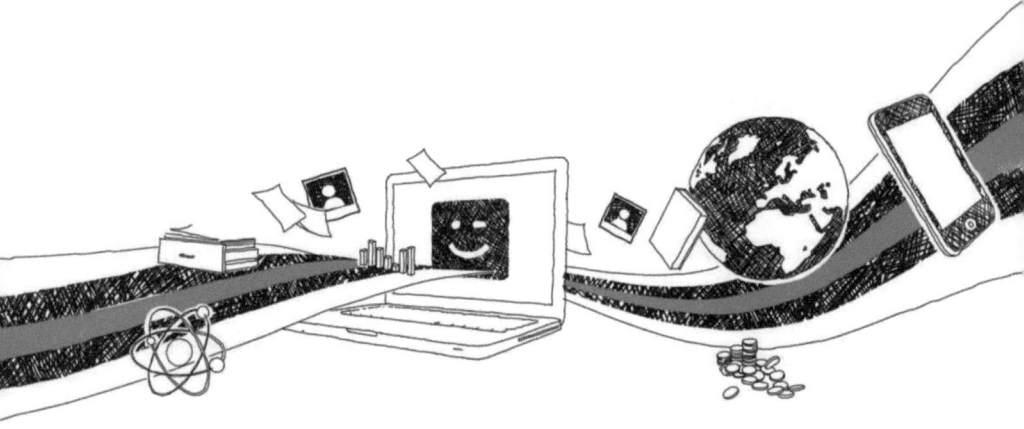

- We will publish your bachelor's and
  master's thesis, essays and papers

- Your own eBook and book -
  sold worldwide in all relevant shops

- Earn money with each sale

Upload your text at www.GRIN.com
and publish for free

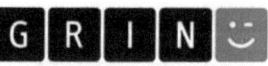